Table of Contents

Understanding Your Carbon Footprint

In the realm of sustainable living, understanding the carbon footprint is foundational. This measure reflects the total greenhouse gases emitted directly and indirectly by human actions. Grasping its scope is crucial not only for fostering awareness but also for empowering individuals to enact meaningful change. As one delves into the nuts and bolts of carbon footprint calculations, the journey begins to demystify the abstract concept, turning it into something personally significant and actionable.

Imagine your daily routine as a web of interconnected decisions. From the moment you brew your morning coffee to the commute you take and the clothes you wear, every choice contributes to your overall carbon output. Though seemingly small on their own, these decisions accumulate over time, forming a larger environmental impact. Understanding these connections is the first step toward adopting a more conscious, eco-friendly lifestyle.

Transportation stands as a notable player in personal carbon emissions. Vehicles powered by fossil fuels release a considerable amount of carbon dioxide into the atmosphere. As the global population continues to grow, the reliance on personal cars compounds the challenge. By recognizing the weight of these decisions, we open the door to exploring alternative travel options that align better with sustainable living goals.

Energy consumption forms another critical part of the carbon footprint equation. From the electricity that powers your home to the devices you use, each energy source can vary greatly in its environmental impact. By choosing renewable energy providers or implementing energy-saving practices, individuals can make significant reductions in their personal emissions without necessarily sacrificing comfort or convenience.

Our consumption habits, often overlooked, play a pivotal role in shaping carbon emissions. The production, transportation, and disposal of goods all contribute to the total carbon footprint. By opting for mindful purchasing and reducing waste, one can lower their environmental impact. These conscious changes not only benefit the planet but also foster a more intentional and rewarding lifestyle.

As we plant the seeds for understanding individual impacts on global emissions, the coming pages will guide you through practical, measurable steps. Together, we will explore how small, intentional changes can collectively lead to substantial reductions in carbon output, paving the way for a sustainable future that is within reach for everyone.

In the quest to grasp your carbon footprint, it's essential to start with an awareness of consumption patterns in electricity. Simple actions like turning off lights when leaving a room or unplugging unused devices can gradually decrease energy consumption. Moreover, investing in programmable thermostats allows for optimized heating and cooling schedules, reducing the need for constant energy use. Such measures not only lessen your carbon output but also offer financial savings over time.

Transitioning to alternative energy sources further amplifies the impact. Solar panels, for instance, provide a renewable resource that can power a household, significantly lowering reliance on carbon-intensive electricity. Similarly, choosing providers that offer green energy plans contributes to a cleaner demand-supply chain. While such changes may initially seem costly or daunting, they can be incremental and tailored to fit individual circumstances.

When considering transportation, the shift from driving alone to carpooling or using public transit stands as a meaningful step toward reducing emissions. Walking or cycling for short trips not only cuts down on fuel consumption but also promotes personal health and well-being. If vehicle maintenance is a necessity, routine check-ups aligned with ensuring fuel efficiency also contribute positively.

Dietary habits, though often underestimated, significantly influence one's carbon footprint. Opting for locally sourced produce minimizes the need for long-distance transportation that fuels emissions. A preference for plant-based meals, even a few times a week, effectively curtails the exhaustive resources required for meat production. Being mindful of these choices resonates far beyond personal health, echoing in broader ecological conservation.

Waste management is another focal point in carbon footprint reduction. Practicing recycling and composting reclaims materials that would otherwise contribute to landfill emissions. A keen eye on purchasing decisions—favoring products with minimal packaging and opting for reusable items—furthers a commitment to reducing wastage.

Understanding your carbon footprint is not a one-time endeavor but an ongoing journey. It's about continuously re-evaluating and adjusting your lifestyle choices to align with personal and environmental values. As we traverse these initial steps, the knowledge gained equips us to delve deeper into more nuanced aspects of sustainable living, setting the stage for the transformative strategies that follow. These small adjustments lead to larger systemic practices, the exploration of which will continue to unfold.

As we wrap up our exploration of carbon footprints, it's vital to remember that the knowledge gained is only as useful as the actions that follow. Understanding your carbon footprint is less about achieving perfection and more about striving for consciousness in everyday decisions. Change begins with small, manageable steps, gradually leading to more significant shifts that align with sustainable living.

Consider your home environment as a canvas for change. By implementing straightforward measures such as using energy-efficient bulbs and insulating your home, you bring about a dual benefit of reducing both carbon emissions and household costs. Tying these improvements into habitual routines cultivates a sense of responsibility and accomplishment, encouraging further initiatives.

Exploring the cultural and social dynamics surrounding consumption can uncover additional pathways to lower your footprint. Joining local farmers' markets, for instance, supports community-based agriculture and ensures access to fresh, sustainably sourced foods. These communal engagements not only sustain an eco-conscious diet but also build meaningful connections with those who share similar values.

Moreover, transportation alternatives are not confined to personal gains; they ripple outwards, influencing public awareness and policy. By choosing to walk or cycle, you contribute to the growing demand for infrastructure that supports non-motorized transit. Advocacy for improved public transport can also elevate accessibility, making sustainable choices more viable for others.

Engaging in conversations around these changes amplifies their impact. Sharing personal experiences with peers fosters a collective understanding and pushes the boundaries of individual efforts. Encouragement comes not just from witnessing shared successes but also from learning from setbacks, enriching the journey toward sustainable living.

Ultimately, the pursuit of sustainability is a lifelong commitment, an ever-evolving response to the intricate interplay of human activities and the natural world. By continually refining your understanding and actions related to carbon emissions, you become an advocate for the planet—one decision, one step at a time.

Reducing Energy Consumption

Embracing energy efficiency begins at home, where the cumulative impact of our choices can inspire broader ecological benefits. The journey to reducing energy consumption doesn't necessitate grand alterations; instead, it focuses on small, thoughtful adjustments that seamlessly integrate into daily life. Recognizing the value of energy conservation not only moves us closer to sustainable goals but also brings tangible savings, enhancing our quality of life in the process.

The first step in reducing energy usage is an evaluation of household appliances. Older models, though functional, often lack the energy efficiency seen in newer designs. Where possible, consider upgrades to items labeled with the Energy Star certification, which signifies adherence to stringent efficiency standards. These appliances operate using less power without compromising performance, thereby reducing both your carbon footprint and utility bills.

In conjunction to upgrading appliances, adopting smart home technology offers another layer of control over energy use. Devices such as smart thermostats, which adjust temperatures based on your household's schedule, ensure heating and cooling systems operate only when needed. This not only lowers consumption but also maintains comfort, illustrating that technology and sustainability can comfortably coexist.

Daily habits play an equally critical role in curbing energy consumption. Simple actions, such as turning off lights in unoccupied rooms or bathing in cooler water, may seem inconsequential individually but produce significant reductions collectively. Moreover, integrating these small changes into established routines encourages more mindful energy use across all areas of life, extending beyond the confines of our homes.

Lighting constitutes a substantial portion of residential energy use, making it a prime candidate for optimization. Replacing incandescent bulbs with LED alternatives presents an effective strategy for lowering energy expenditure. LEDs not only draw less power but also have a longer lifespan, offering dual benefits for both the environment and household costs over time.

As these strategies take root, it is important to remain open to adaptation. Energy efficiency is ever-evolving, and by staying informed of new technologies and practices, one can continuously refine their approach. The pursuit of energy reduction invites not just immediate changes but fosters a mindset of perpetual improvement, setting the stage for continued exploration in sustainable living practices.

One often underrated area where energy savings can be realized is the insulation within a home. Proper insulation acts as a barrier to heat loss and heat gain, depending on the season. By ensuring that walls, roofs, and floors are well-insulated, homeowners can significantly reduce the dependence on heating and cooling systems. This not only diminishes energy use but also creates a more consistent indoor climate, enhancing overall comfort.

Investing in energy-efficient windows is another impactful strategy. These windows are designed to limit the transfer of heat, keeping warm air inside during the winter and cool air during the summer. Despite the upfront cost, the long-term savings on energy bills, along with increased property value, make this an appealing option. Coupled with window coverings such as blinds or curtains, they provide added layers of insulation, further enhancing their efficiency.

Water heating is a significant energy expense in most households, yet it often goes unnoticed. Adjusting water heater settings to a lower temperature conserves energy without substantially affecting everyday activities. Installing a solar water heater could also be an excellent alternative, harnessing renewable energy to meet your household's hot water needs. These small adjustments contribute to a broader strategy for energy efficiency, aligning economic benefits with environmental stewardship.

To maximize the efficiency of your heating and cooling systems, regular maintenance is vital. Ensuring that filters are replaced, ducts are sealed, and systems are properly calibrated enhances performance while reducing unnecessary energy consumption. Preventive care prolongs the lifespan of equipment, securing your investment and ensuring that your home remains an energy-efficient hub.

Programs that offer energy audits or consultations can provide further insight. These assessments identify specific areas for improvement and tailor solutions according to individual needs. They detail steps for enhanced efficiency, sometimes even suggesting available rebates or incentives that offset costs. Engaging in these opportunities reveals hidden efficiencies, streamlining the journey towards sustainable living.

As these practical steps become part of the norm, they lay the groundwork for more comprehensive energy solutions. Innovations such as home energy management systems can be explored to further optimize consumption patterns. These systems provide real-time data and control, enabling efficient responses to energy needs as they arise. By integrating these tools, the household transforms into an ecosystem of sustainability, ready for future advancements.

As we conclude our exploration of energy consumption, it's crucial to address the often-overlooked impact of phantom energy use. Devices that remain plugged in, even when not actively in use, continue to draw power. This subtle yet persistent drain can be mitigated by utilizing power strips to easily disconnect multiple appliances or by choosing smart plugs that cut off energy to devices when they're not needed. Such small adjustments represent effortless ways to curb unnecessary consumption and champion mindful energy use.

Thermal mass, an often underutilized concept, can further bolster energy efficiency. Materials such as stone, brick, and concrete naturally absorb and retain heat, which can be a boon during winter months. By incorporating elements with high thermal mass into the design of your home, you can stabilize indoor temperatures without increasing reliance on heating systems—an ingenious blend of architectural wisdom and sustainability.

Adding renewable energy sources into your energy reduction strategy is an enriching endeavor. Supplement your household's power needs with small-scale wind turbines or solar panels if feasible. These additions not only decrease dependency on grid energy but also promote self-sufficiency, aligning seamlessly with the ethos of sustainable living. For those not yet ready to fully invest in solar, community solar initiatives offer a way to share in the benefits of renewable power collaboratively.

Engagement in community-based energy programs further extends your influence. By participating, you promote wider adoption of sustainable practices and foster connections with others committed to similar goals. Collaboration within these networks cultivates a shared understanding of energy conservation challenges and solutions, enriching your own journey while contributing to collective progress.

In bringing it all together, gradual changes rooted in awareness cut significantly through the tangle of energy use, leaving a path towards a more harmonious and sustainable lifestyle. The benefits are tangible—lower utility bills and reduced carbon emissions—yet the ripple effects are profound, reshaping the way we perceive and engage with our environment. Taking proactive steps to reduce energy consumption is a practice of empowerment, transforming your living space into a testament of sustainability that genuinely inspires.

As these principles permeate your daily life, they serve as reminders of the broader narrative of conservation and respect for our planet. With every informed choice, from leveraging technology to fostering community spirit, you become part of a larger movement committed to safeguarding our natural world for future generations. These efforts, though beginning at home, undoubtedly extend beyond, creating a culture of responsibility and sustainability.

Sustainable Transportation

Transportation choices profoundly influence our carbon footprint, offering an opportunity to shift toward more sustainable models. For many, the traditional car remains a staple of daily life, yet its environmental costs invite reconsideration. As cities grow and adapt, so too must our transit habits. Embracing alternatives that promote sustainability becomes not only beneficial but necessary.

Walking and cycling represent the most accessible forms of eco-friendly transportation. These modes not only cut down on carbon emissions but also foster health benefits and community engagement. Urban landscapes increasingly accommodate pedestrians and cyclists, with dedicated pathways and bike-share programs making active travel more attractive. By choosing these options, we contribute to decongesting roadways and improving air quality.

Public transportation holds a unique position in the sustainable travel sphere. Buses, trains, and trams, when widely utilized, significantly reduce the number of individual vehicles on the road. Investing in public transit systems manifests in decreased emissions, less traffic congestion, and better connectivity across regions. Learning to navigate these networks effectively can be both liberating and environmentally considerate.

Carpooling provides another layer of sustainability to car travel. Sharing rides not only reduces fuel consumption and emissions per person but also creates opportunities for social interaction, making commuting a more shared experience. Digital platforms that facilitate ride-sharing further simplify the process, enhancing accessibility and convenience.

For those considering vehicle ownership, the advent of electric and hybrid vehicles offers a path toward cleaner technology. These vehicles use renewable energy sources to reduce dependency on fossil fuels, aligning personal mobility with environmental goals. While upfront costs may be higher, the long-term benefits in terms of fuel savings and reduced emissions justify the investment.

Exploring these sustainable transportation options requires informed decision-making. As we progress, the focus will be on understanding the broader networks and infrastructures that facilitate these choices, paving the way for innovations that support a lower-carbon future. Transitioning thoughtfully can reshape our individual impact and collective responsibility in transportation.

Embracing sustainable transportation involves more than merely choosing alternative methods; it's about rethinking our relationship with movement. Consider the rhythm of daily routines—each choice, from short errands to longer commutes, presents a chance to opt for eco-friendly alternatives. By consciously prioritizing sustainable options, we reshape not only personal habits but also broader urban landscapes.

The essence of walking and cycling lies in their simplicity and accessibility. These forms of transportation require minimal investment while returning profound benefits. As cities continue to invest in infrastructure that supports these methods, the ease of connecting with nature and local environments grows. Streetscapes, once dominated by vehicles, transform into vibrant spaces, fostering a stronger sense of community.

Public transportation scales accessibility across diverse demographics, building connectivity that extends beyond urban centers. Reliability and efficiency in transit systems not only reduce emissions but also present significant cost savings. As cities innovate, offering both traditional and modern transit solutions like electric buses, commuters are invited to participate in a cleaner, shared future.

The conversation around carpooling often centers on its practicality, yet it also serves as a potent tool for collective action. By consolidating journeys, individuals contribute to reducing traffic burden and fuel consumption. Technology-driven platforms enhance the ability to coordinate among commuters, making it easier to align schedules and share resources.

For those exploring vehicle ownership, electric and hybrid vehicles stand as a testament to technological advancement and environmental consciousness. These vehicles mark a pivotal shift in how personal transportation can contribute to carbon reduction goals. While the transition may entail initial adjustments, the potential return on investment—both ecological and financial—is compelling.

As each transportation choice ripples outward, the impact multiplies. Collective movement towards sustainable options influences infrastructure development, policy-making, and public advocacy. In choosing these paths, individuals contribute to crafting an ecosystem of transportation that aligns with sustainable living, setting in motion possibilities for innovation and growth.

Choosing sustainable transportation is akin to embracing a shift in perspective, emphasizing simplicity and interconnectedness. As individuals, we hold the reins to transform our transit habits into purposeful choices that reflect a commitment to a healthier planet. Opting for walking or cycling whenever feasible embodies the ethos of minimal impact while engendering personal wellness and a deeper appreciation of our surroundings.

Transitioning to public transit entails more than just geographic exploration; it's about harmonious coexistence within shared spaces. As we traverse cityscapes, buses and trains become conduits for reducing collective emissions. By investing time in understanding these networks, we align our routines with an eco-friendly lifestyle that redefines convenience through sustainability.

Car-sharing has emerged as a modern solution to traditional vehicle ownership, capitalizing on community cooperation while minimizing resource usage. By connecting with like-minded commuters, we reduce our carbon footprints and create bonds over shared experiences. The simplicity of car-sharing is its strength, delivering practical ease without extra environmental cost.

When contemplating vehicle ownership, delving into the realm of electric and hybrid cars can spark transformative change. These vehicles challenge the status quo, aligning innovation with conservation. As technology advances, the barriers to adopting these eco-friendly alternatives diminish, inviting a broader embrace that transcends generational divides.

Navigating transportation choices is a journey in itself, laden with opportunities to marry practicality and purpose. As infrastructure increasingly accommodates these shifts, individuals can take part in driving policy and promoting sustainable reforms. This empowerment on the road fosters a sense of ownership over environmental impact, setting the stage for continual progress.

By consciously integrating sustainable transportation into daily life, we not only refine our individual carbon profiles but also inspire collective movement toward resilience. In each small decision lies a ripple effect that reverberates beyond our personal paths, crafting a narrative of change that has the potential to reshape societal norms for generations to come.

Eco-Friendly Food Choices

In the quest for sustainability, the food choices we make hold significant sway over environmental health and personal well-being. The journey begins with an awareness of how food production contributes to ecological strain. Industrial agriculture, while feeding millions, often leaves a massive carbon footprint due to the energy-intensive processes involved. Shifting towards eco-friendly food choices can mitigate these impacts while enhancing nutritional value.

Adopting a plant-based diet stands as a cornerstone of sustainable eating. Plants require fewer resources compared to animal agriculture, making vegetarian and vegan meals highly effective in reducing environmental pressure. This dietary shift doesn't mandate a complete overhaul but rather encourages the exploration of plant-centric dishes, highlighting their diversity and culinary potential.

Minimizing food waste is another powerful lever in sustainable living. Waste occurs at every stage of the food supply chain, with household waste accounting for a significant portion. By planning meals thoughtfully and storing produce correctly, individuals can cut down on waste, keeping both the pantry and conscience clear.

Understanding food labels is crucial for informed, sustainable consumption. Labels often offer insights into the origins and contents of products, guiding decisions that align with personal values and environmental considerations. Knowledge of certifications like organic or fair trade can further inform choices, ensuring they meet ethical standards.

Embracing local and seasonal foods not only supports regional farmers but also reduces the need for transportation, decreasing the carbon footprint associated with food miles. Consuming what's abundant and fresh in your area fosters a connection to the land and its cycles, enriching your culinary experience and sense of place.

As we delve deeper into the nuances of sustainable eating, it becomes clear that each meal is an opportunity to weave environmental stewardship into daily life. Through mindful selections and a deeper appreciation of food's journey from farm to table, sustainable living becomes a flavorful and rewarding pursuit.

The journey towards eco-friendly food choices begins with a willingness to explore the abundant variety within plant-based eating. Embracing vegetables, legumes, nuts, and grains as staples can transform not only meals but also our relationship with food. Beyond the environmental benefits, these ingredients offer diverse flavors and textures, inviting creativity in the kitchen. Transitioning to a plant-centered diet can be gradual—each substitution contributes positively towards a more sustainable lifestyle.

Another critical aspect of sustainable food practices is the reduction of waste, which necessitates a proactive approach. Implementing a waste reduction strategy starts with planning meals that utilize ingredients fully and repurposing leftovers creatively. Storing food properly extends its freshness, while composting any scraps closes the loop, returning nutrients to the earth. This cycle of mindful consumption and waste management fosters a holistic connection to our food sources.

Food labeling, often a source of confusion, can serve as a tool for making conscientious choices. By decoding the information provided on packaging, such as origin and certifications, we gain insight into the ethics and sustainability of our purchases. Understanding what terms like "organic" or "non-GMO" entail supports informed decisions tailored to personal values and environmental impact. This awareness empowers consumers to align their buying habits with sustainable principles.

Local and seasonal eating intertwines with sustainable practices by aligning consumption with the natural rhythms of agriculture. Frequenting farmers' markets or joining community-supported agriculture programs ensures access to fresh produce with a minimal carbon footprint. This practice nurtures local economies and encourages biodiversity in crop production. Celebrating local flavors and seasonal abundance deepens our appreciation for the environment and its gifts.

Incorporating these strategies into daily life not only boosts personal health but also bolsters ecological conservation efforts. Choosing eco-friendly food options demonstrates a commitment to reducing harm and preserving resources. As our understanding of sustainable eating matures, it becomes possible to engage deeper in the narrative of interconnectedness between people and the planet.

This chapter continues its exploration into how simple dietary adjustments can serve as powerful catalysts for change. By mindfully considering the origins and impacts of our food, we cultivate a profound respect for the intricate food networks that sustain us. The journey towards sustainable eating invites us to savor each meal as an opportunity to act in harmony with the world around us. This mindset will guide the next phases of our sustainable living exploration, enriching our understanding and implementation of eco-conscious choices.

Incorporating a plant-based diet can significantly lower your personal carbon footprint, thus supporting environmental efforts. Introducing variety with items like lentils, beans, and tofu enriches your meals while contributing less to agricultural emissions. Beyond reducing meat consumption, this shift encourages biodiversity by increasing demand for diverse crops, which benefits both the land and local ecosystems.

As we cultivate these new habits, food waste emerges as a key focus for sustainability. The choices made at the grocery store ripple into kitchen practices—planning portions and embracing leftovers prevent food from ending up in landfills, where they release methane, a potent greenhouse gas. Composting non-edible scraps not only reduces waste but enriches soil, closing the loop in the food cycle.

Empowering yourself with knowledge about food labels plays an essential role in making conscious consumption choices. Beyond the marketing slogans, labels reveal crucial information about the sources and methods of production. Understanding these can guide us towards products that reflect sustainable, ethical, and health-conscious values, ultimately influencing industry practices.

Eating locally and seasonally bolsters the link between consumers and their immediate environment. By embracing the produce available within our regions, we diminish the environmental toll associated with long-distance transportation. Additionally, supporting local agriculture fosters sustainable land use and reduces dependency on intensive farming practices that deplete resources.

The journey to sustainable eating is not just about diet; it's a holistic approach to consuming responsibly. This transition invites exploration and creativity, nurturing a deeper connection to the world of food. As we align our dietary habits with environmental consciousness, the ripple effects extend beyond personal health, supporting broader efforts to preserve our planet.

Closing this chapter on eco-friendly food choices, we stand at the threshold of endless possibilities for nurturing both our bodies and the earth. With each mindful decision, we help chart a path towards a more sustainable future, wherein every meal reflects a commitment to ecological responsibility and well-being.

Cultivating Your Own Food

Embarking on the journey of cultivating your own food transforms your relationship with what you eat. It offers a direct line to food production and fosters a connection to the cycles of nature. This endeavor does not require sprawling lands; rather, it's about utilizing whatever space you have, be it a backyard, a small patio, or a sunny windowsill. By taking these steps, you not only gain control over your food quality but also contribute to ecological sustainability.

The first step in this venture is understanding your available space and resources. Evaluate where you can plant, considering sunlight, wind exposure, and the potential for soil or containers. Each variable influences what grows best, whether you're eyeing tender herbs or hardy root vegetables. This planning stage ensures that your efforts will flourish, tailored to your unique environment. Beginning with simple crops can ease the learning curve and offer quick rewards.

Urban gardening often conjures images of vast vegetable patches, yet it can start simply with container gardening. Using pots or recycled containers, you can cultivate a variety of produce, even in the smallest of spaces. Herbs like basil or cilantro, along with vegetables such as tomatoes and peppers, thrive in confined conditions. This approach allows flexibility in arrangement and movement, accommodating for seasonal changes or relocations.

Part of successful cultivation includes nurturing the foundation—your soil. A rich, well-balanced medium provides the essential nutrients for plant growth. If natural soil is not an option, a mixture of potting soil, compost, and organic matter serves as a robust alternative. Regularly refreshing your soil with homemade compost not only enriches it but also recycles food waste effectively, enhancing both plant health and ecological balance.

Composting, an integral aspect of sustainable gardening, turns kitchen leftovers into valuable soil amendments. Initiating a compost system, whether a simple bin or a more sophisticated tumbler, diverts organic waste from landfills. Over time, this matter breaks down into nutrient-rich compost, ready to boost your garden's resilience. Engaging with this cycle introduces a rewarding dimension to food production, fostering awareness of the complete loop from seed to table and back again.

Above all, cultivating your food is a practice in patience and observance. As you nurture seedlings to maturity, you witness firsthand the impact of weather, water, and care. This process becomes a living tutorial in resilience and adaptation. Each harvest underscores the rewards of your efforts, providing fresh produce imbued with the satisfaction of self-reliance and the knowledge that you are contributing positively to the environment. As with any journey, the experiences gathered become stepping stones to further exploration and expansion in sustainable living.

Embracing home gardening offers an incredible opportunity to connect with nature in a deeply personal way. The joy of nurturing plants from seed to harvest brings immense satisfaction, integrating the rhythms of growth into your everyday life. Whether you have plenty of outdoor space or are confined to a balcony, even the smallest garden can provide a bounty of fresh produce. Your edible landscape not only brightens your surroundings but also fills your table with fresh eats cultivated by your own hands.

Maximize limited areas with vertical gardening, a savvy solution when ground real estate is restricted. Utilize trellises, wall planters, and hanging baskets to grow a variety of crops like peas and beans that naturally climb. This approach makes efficient use of space while adding an aesthetic dimension to your garden. Vertical gardening allows for efficient irrigation practices as well, ensuring that plants receive adequate water without wastage.

Caring for your fledgling garden involves a basic understanding of companion planting, an age-old technique to naturally deter pests and enhance growth. By planting certain species together, you can create a mutually beneficial environment that reduces the need for chemical interventions. For instance, marigolds can draw aphids away from your delicate veggies, while the strong scent of herbs like mint and rosemary can deter garden nuisances.

Attention to watering practices ensures plant vitality. It's critical to recognize the specific hydration needs of different crops to avoid over or under-watering. Investing in a drip irrigation system can be a wise move; these systems provide a steady, measured supply of water directly to the root zones. This not only conserves water but can also prevent soil erosion and nutrient loss, nurturing a thriving garden ecosystem.

Sunlight exposure is another essential factor in planting success. By observing how light moves across your space during the day, you can better position plants according to their sunlight requirements. Leafy greens like spinach and lettuce prefer cooler, shaded spots, whereas sun-loving species, such as tomatoes and peppers, thrive in direct sunlight. Tailoring the placement of plants optimizes growth potential and encourages robust yields.

As your garden matures, it becomes a testament to sustainable practices, blending personal wellness with environmental responsibility. With each passing season, lessons learned from successes and challenges in the garden deepen your understanding, cultivating not only plants but also a more sustainable approach to daily living. As you persist in this rewarding journey, every new sprout celebrates your dedication and reflects the promise of nature's generosity.

As you embark on cultivating your own food, begin with an exploration of what you wish to grow. Consider your dietary preferences and the climate of your region. Opt for plants that thrive locally, making the most of their natural resilience. This thoughtful selection is foundational as it ensures your garden aligns with both your ecological conditions and your culinary desires.

Assessing the type of soil you have is crucial, as it forms the bedrock for growth. Rich, loamy soil supports a wide range of plants, providing essential nutrients and excellent drainage. If your natural soil needs enhancement, organic matter like compost and mulch can transform its quality over time. Regularly supplementing soil with these materials fortifies plant health, optimizing your garden's productivity.

Seeds or seedlings, the initial choice depends on your patience and experience. Direct sowing seeds can be a cost-effective method and allows you to witness every stage of life, from sprout to bloom. On the other hand, acquiring seedlings accelerates the process, offering a head start in cultivation. Regardless of the choice, ensure seeds are sourced from reputable vendors, promoting biodiversity and quality.

The ecological benefits of home gardening extend beyond just harvesting food. It attracts beneficial insects such as pollinators, enriching the local environment's biodiversity. Bees and butterflies play a pivotal role in the health of your garden, enhancing growth through their natural interactions. Create habitats for these allies by including flowering plants among your crops, encouraging their vital presence.

Throughout this journey, adapt to the challenges and embrace the lessons nature offers. Weather fluctuations, pest invasions, and unexpected growth cycles teach resilience and adaptability. Each difficulty met cultivates a deeper bond with your environment and enhances your skillset, preparing you for future gardening endeavors.

Ultimately, as you savor the fruits of your labor, you'll appreciate not just the fresh produce but also the knowledge and insight gained. Cultivating food at home is a testament to self-reliance and sustainability, encapsulating a journey where every plant speaks of care, effort, and a commitment to the earth's well-being.

Minimalism and Sustainable Consumption

In a world driven by the constant hum of consumerism, minimalism offers a refreshing approach to living more intentionally. It's not about scarcity, but rather about discerning the essentials and shedding the superfluous. As we explore this lifestyle, we're invited to scrutinize our consumption patterns and uncover the depths of fulfillment that simplicity can bring.

Minimalism encourages us to redefine our relationship with material possessions. By recognizing the difference between need and want, we can navigate our consumer choices with greater clarity. This introspection reveals not only the physical clutter that surrounds us but also the mental clutter weighing on our minds.

The impact of fast fashion, a sector notorious for its rapid cycles and immense waste, serves as a poignant example of unsustainable consumption. The fleeting nature of trends necessitates frequent purchases, contributing to overfilled closets and overflowing landfills. This realization prompts reflection on our sartorial decisions and inspires shifts toward sustainable fashion choices.

Equally concerning is the phenomenon of planned obsolescence, where products are designed with an intentionally limited lifespan. This practice fuels the cycle of consumerism, pushing us toward continuous upgrading rather than repair. By resisting this model and opting for longevity and quality, we reclaim our agency against needless consumption.

Adopting a minimalist mindset is not a one-time transformation but a sustained journey of mindful acquisition. It involves a deliberate approach to gifting and receiving, focusing on experiences rather than material goods. As we embrace this philosophy, we cultivate a life enriched by purpose rather than possession.

As we delve deeper into the practical steps of minimalism, we'll explore methods to responsibly dispose of excess and create spaces that reflect simplicity and intentionality. This unfolding journey challenges us to rethink our consumer habits and embrace a lifestyle that aligns with sustainable values, setting the groundwork for a new perspective on living.

To begin embracing a minimalist lifestyle, it's essential to start with a clear understanding of your personal consumption patterns. Pause and assess each item you own: consider its purpose and the joy it brings. This practice, often referred to as a "possessions audit," helps identify items that genuinely enrich your life versus those that clutter it. By recognizing the excess, you can begin to pare down your belongings, keeping only what is truly meaningful and necessary.

Once you embark on minimizing your possessions, organization becomes key. As you declutter, categorize items into those you'll keep, donate, or responsibly dispose of. This method not only creates physical space but also instills a sense of mental clarity. As you go through this process, aim to focus on quality over quantity in future purchases, aligning each acquisition with your core values and needs.

The allure of fast fashion often poses a challenge to sustainability goals. To counter this, explore the realm of conscious fashion, where thoughtful purchases support ethical production and longer-lasting use. Consider building a versatile wardrobe with timeless, well-crafted pieces that withstand fleeting trends. In doing so, you can significantly reduce waste and acknowledge the environmental footprints of your choices.

Mindful consumption extends beyond clothing to every aspect of life. When purchasing new items, question their long-term utility and environmental impact. Opt for products that offer longevity rather than quick fixes, thus resisting the cycle of planned obsolescence. By making deliberate choices, you champion sustainability and alleviate the burden on natural resources.

As you adopt a minimalist approach, gifts and celebrations offer unique opportunities to align with these principles. Prioritize experiences over physical gifts, such as sharing memorable activities with loved ones. This shift encourages deeper connections and reduces clutter, fostering a more meaningful way to participate in special occasions.

This ongoing journey of minimalism invites continuous reflection and adaptability. Each decision, whether small or significant, reinforces a commitment to living with intention. As you cultivate simplicity in consumption, you lay a foundation for a more sustainable, fulfilling life, poised to embrace the contents of the subsequent pages with newfound clarity.

Embracing minimalism begins with a conscious decision to detoxify your environment from unnecessary items. Start small, perhaps with a single room or space, and systematically assess its contents. Each object's value is measured not just by its utility but by the joy or function it provides. This process of decluttering is not simply about getting rid of things; it's an exercise in self-awareness and realistic assessment of needs versus wants.

Transitioning to a life of minimalism includes cultivating habits that discourage impulsive buying. When considering a new purchase, ask yourself whether it serves a genuine purpose or merely satisfies a momentary desire. By practicing patience, you allow time to evaluate the true necessity of an item, promoting intentional consumption that aligns with your minimalist goals.

The fashion industry often seduces with its rapid cycles and new trends, making it a primary focus for minimalist changes. Instead of chasing stylish whims, invest in timeless pieces that stand the test of time. Seek out sustainable brands that prioritize quality and ethics, reducing the fashion footprint and nurturing a more thoughtful wardrobe.

Minimalism isn't purely about physical possessions; it extends to digital consumption as well. Evaluate your digital life—unsubscribe from unnecessary newsletters, organize files, and streamline apps. This creates virtual breathing space and reduces the stress of digital clutter. By managing both physical and digital realms, you enhance mental clarity and contentment.

Mindful disposal of belongings plays an integral role in minimalism. Consider donating to local charities or recycling, reducing the burden on landfills and supporting a circular economy. Developing a habit of thoughtful disposal ensures that you handle possessions responsibly even at the end of their lifecycle.

As we close this reflection on minimalism, remember that embracing simplicity is a pathway to enhanced focus and fulfillment. By fostering mindfulness in consumption, you build a life enriched by experience rather than accumulation. This mindset not only nurtures personal well-being but also contributes to a sustainable future.

Waste Reduction and Recycling

In our modern world, waste management has emerged as a crucial element of sustainable living. It's not just about throwing things away—it's about understanding the lifecycle of our possessions and transforming how we interact with them. This shift in mindset can lead to not only environmental benefits but also personal and community improvement. As you embark on this journey, envision a lifestyle where waste is minimized and resources are valued.

Achieving a zero-waste lifestyle begins with a fundamental reevaluation of the materials we bring into our lives. This requires a conscious effort to refuse unnecessary items, reduce consumption, and prioritize sustainability. By making deliberate choices about what we buy and how we use it, we can drastically cut down what ends up in our trash cans. This approach doesn't demand immediate perfection but rather gradual, consistent effort toward waste reduction.

Recycling responsibly is a cornerstone of managing waste effectively. It's about more than just tossing items into the recycling bin; it involves understanding the specifics of what can and cannot be recycled in your local area. Comprehending these guidelines ensures that materials are properly processed, avoiding contamination and inefficiencies in recycling facilities. This diligence in sorting reinforces the overall efficacy of recycling efforts.

Upcycling offers a creative twist on the traditional concept of recycling. By reimagining the value of old or worn items, you can transform them into something new and functional. This practice not only diverts waste from landfills but also stimulates creativity and innovation. Whether transforming glass jars into stylish storage solutions or repurposing old clothes into unique textiles, upcycling instills a sense of achievement and ecological mindfulness.

At the heart of waste reduction lies the practice of thoughtful disposal. Composting organic waste allows for the natural decomposition of food scraps and yard debris, returning valuable nutrients to the soil. This process not only diminishes landfill contributions but also enriches gardens and green spaces, creating a full-circle approach to waste management. Engaging with composting can enhance your connection to nature's cycles and bolster efforts in creating a more sustainable home environment.

As this chapter unfolds, it will delve deeper into strategies that integrate seamlessly into everyday life, effectively minimizing your environmental footprint. These practices, while simple, align with broader initiatives dedicated to preserving our planet. The focus remains on continuous improvement and adapting strategies that meet the evolving needs of our society and environment. In this journey of waste reduction and recycling, the smallest actions can lead to significant change, influencing both your immediate surroundings and the larger global narrative of sustainability.

Reconsidering traditional waste disposal habits opens the door to a more sustainable lifestyle where each decision influences broader environmental outcomes. Essential to this shift is the art of refusing—an intentional act of rejecting items that contribute to waste. This involves saying no to single-use plastics, unnecessary packaging, and disposable products that offer fleeting convenience at the cost of sustainability.

In tandem with refusal, waste reduction emphasizes mindfulness in consumption. It encourages us to purchase with purpose, choosing quality over quantity. By prioritizing durable, reusable, and repairable goods, we not only curb waste but also foster a culture of preservation and thoughtful use. This approach invites us to see the value in what we already own, prolonging the lifecycle of products and reducing the need for frequent replacements.

Transitioning to a lifestyle that embraces recycling requires a keen understanding of local recycling guidelines. This means familiarizing yourself with what materials are accepted, ensuring that they are free of contaminants, and separating them accordingly. By doing so, you improve the efficiency of recycling processes, contributing to a more robust system that sustains the community and reduces landfill overflow.

Upcycling stands as a creative pillar within waste management practices. It transforms items poised for disposal into something innovative and functional. Engaging in upcycling projects can range from simple endeavors, like turning old magazines into vibrant plant pots, to more complex undertakings, such as crafting furniture from reclaimed wood. This inventive approach not only conserves resources but also enhances personal creativity and resourcefulness.

Composting seamlessly integrates into waste reduction efforts by managing organic matter sustainably. Starting a compost bin, whether indoors with a vermiculture system or outdoors with a traditional heap, captures food scraps and yard waste, returning them to the earth in the form of nutrient-rich soil amendments. This practice closes the loop in waste disposal, minimizing contributions to methane-emitting landfills and enriching garden ecosystems.

Embracing a zero-waste mindset transforms how we engage with our surroundings, revealing the interconnections between personal habits and ecological health. As we incorporate these techniques into daily routines, we shift from mere consumers to active participants in the sustainability journey. Each small step builds momentum for larger changes, culminating in a lifestyle that reveres resources and champions environmental renewal.

Equipped with the understanding that waste reduction starts at home, let's explore tangible actions that reshape our waste management habits. Begin by scrutinizing household consumption with a strategic eye. Opt for products in bulk to minimize packaging, and choose items that come in recyclable or compostable materials whenever possible. This proactive approach not only decreases immediate waste but fosters long-term habits that champion sustainability.

Find ways to reimagine everyday objects through creative repurposing, unlocking the hidden potential within items often discarded. Simple kitchen jars transform into stylish storage solutions, while worn-out T-shirts can be reborn as cleaning rags. This practice of upcycling propels a shift in mindset, seeing value in the overlooked and promoting a cycle of renewal rather than disposal.

An essential part of cultivating a zero-waste lifestyle involves developing systems for proper sorting and disposing of waste at home. Install clearly labeled recycling bins to encourage correct disposal and minimize contamination. Understand the nuances of local recycling programs to ensure compliance and maximization of recycling efforts. By establishing structured routines, we create an environment where sustainability becomes second nature.

On a community level, participating in organized cleanup events highlights the collective responsibility in waste management. Such activities not only beautify shared spaces but inspire widespread awareness about the impact of carelessly discarded waste. By engaging in these communal efforts, individuals contribute to transformative change and reinforce shared commitments to sustainability.

Consider the power of advocating for change within your community. Initiatives can range from suggesting policies to reduce single-use plastics to organizing workshops on composting and recycling. These collective actions amplify individual efforts and demonstrate the impact of unified voices striving for a cleaner environment.

As we conclude this chapter, remember that embracing a sustainable approach to waste management is a journey paved with learning and adaptation. Every mindful action reinforces the understanding that while global change requires systemic shifts, it begins with the decisions we make in our daily lives. Through purposeful reduction, responsible sorting, and creative repurposing, we forge a path toward a more sustainable future—one choice at a time.

Water Conservation Techniques

In the intricate dance of sustainable living, water conservation stands as a cornerstone of resource management. As the global demand for fresh water soars, individuals have the power to make a significant impact through conscious use and careful stewardship of this precious resource. The journey towards wise water usage begins with a shift in mindset, valuing every drop as part of a shared and finite commodity.\n\nWithin our homes, the opportunities for water savings are abundant. By installing fixtures like low-flow showerheads and faucet aerators, we can drastically reduce the amount of water used without sacrificing utility. These simple adjustments represent a fruitful intersection of technology and sustainability, offering immediate benefits both for the environment and household budgets. Additionally, fixing leaks—often underestimated—plays a pivotal role in curbing water waste. A dripping faucet can waste gallons over time, underscoring the necessity for vigilance and routine maintenance.\n\nBeyond hardware solutions, cultivating water-conscious behaviors can lead to substantial conservation. Shortening shower times, turning off the tap while brushing teeth, and running dishwashers only with full loads are small actions that aggregate into meaningful water savings. Such practices champion mindfulness, encouraging a more thoughtful approach to everyday habits that, collectively, have lasting impacts. As individual efforts coalesce, they ripple into wider ecological benefits and set the stage for scalable change.\n\nOn a broader scale, understanding the global water crisis highlights the urgency of these conservation measures. With growing populations and climate changes exacerbating scarcity, water management emerges as both a local responsibility and a global imperative. By recognizing our personal consumption patterns and adapting them, individuals become pivotal players in addressing larger environmental challenges.\n\nEfforts to conserve water extend beyond personal practices. Engaging with local water-saving initiatives or community workshops can amplify individual actions, fostering a culture of stewardship. These collective endeavors provide forums for sharing knowledge, tips, and strategies, thereby reinforcing a communal commitment to water conservation. Harnessing the power of collective action not only multiplies impact but also strengthens the societal will towards sustainable change.\n\nThis seamless blend of individual and community action underscores the interconnected nature of water conservation. As we peel back the layers of our own water usage, we set the groundwork for a more comprehensive exploration. Subsequent sections will delve into innovative methodologies and emerging technologies, guiding us further along the path of water stewardship. Together, we navigate a path that sustains both our planet and its invaluable water resources.

Embracing water scarcity as a pressing global concern, individuals can start making impactful changes at home. One effective method is the utilization of a rainwater harvesting system. By collecting rainwater from rooftops, you provide an alternative source for watering gardens or flushing toilets. This practice lessens the strain on municipal supplies and reduces the volume of water consumption in daily activities, showcasing environmental mindfulness.

Next, consider the benefits of xeriscaping for outdoor spaces. This landscaping technique involves planting drought-resistant flora, aligning gardening habits with water conservation efforts. These plants require significantly less irrigation while adding beauty and ecological value to the home environment. Xeriscaping not only reduces water use but also fosters habitats for native species, contributing to biodiversity.

In urban settings, forming community partnerships focused on water conservation can magnify your impact. Encourage dialogues with local organizations to develop awareness programs or participate in water conservation competitions. Collaborative efforts to install green infrastructure solutions, like green roofs or permeable pavements, can enhance water absorption and reduce runoff, establishing a community-wide norm of resource-conscious living.

Within your living habits, prioritize the re-use of water wherever possible. Greywater systems, for instance, utilize wastewater from showers and sinks for non-potable uses such as watering lawns. This practice ensures that water is cycled through multiple purposes before discharge, optimizing resource use and aligning daily routines with sustainable intentions.

Education plays a pivotal role in fostering responsible water use. Familiarize yourself with regional water conservation initiatives or attend workshops to hone your water management skills. Share this knowledge within your social circles, encouraging others to adopt similar practices. Spreading awareness about efficient water use can create a ripple effect, transforming consciousness at a societal level.

With these practices, the transition towards a more sustainable water usage strategy becomes concrete and achievable. As we journey further in understanding our water footprint, we lay the groundwork for innovative solutions that await exploration. This shared responsibility paves a path toward maintaining our planet's critical water resources, ensuring their availability for future generations.

Exploring water conservation techniques starts with understanding the broader context of our global water usage. As stewards of our planet's resources, it's essential to recognize how daily activities influence local and global water supplies. By adopting simple yet effective habits, we enhance both environmental stewardship and personal responsibility.

Incorporating water-efficient techniques in personal routines marks a significant step forward. Consider using dishwashers and washing machines only with full loads to maximize water efficiency. Additionally, opting for showers instead of baths can substantially reduce water use, making personal hygiene routines more sustainable. These adjustments not only conserve water but can also lead to noticeable savings on monthly water bills.

On a technological front, smart home systems equipped with water usage monitors provide real-time data and feedback on consumption patterns. These systems identify excessive use or leaks, facilitating prompt action to prevent unnecessary wastage. By investing in such technology, individuals take an active role in managing their water footprint with precision and intention.

Gardening practices also offer opportunities for water savings. Employing mulch around plants helps retain soil moisture, reducing the need for frequent watering. Mulching not only conserves water but also enriches the soil, supporting healthier plant growth in a sustainable manner. This approach aligns gardening efforts with broader conservation goals, ensuring every green space contributes to environmental health.

Furthermore, the community dimension cannot be overstated. By participating in local conservation initiatives, residents contribute to a collective effort that amplifies individual actions. Community workshops and forums provide platforms for sharing strategies and innovations, fostering a culture of shared responsibility for water resources.

As this chapter draws to a close, remember that each drop saved contributes to the broader narrative of conservation. By integrating these practices into your lifestyle, you become part of a wider movement dedicated to preserving one of our planet's most vital resources. Together, through mindful action and continuous learning, we pave the way for a sustainable future where water availability and quality are prioritized for generations to come.

Eco-Conscious Home Design

The concept of an eco-conscious home extends beyond aesthetics, integrating functionality with mindful sustainability. This approach considers the lifecycle of materials, emphasizing natural and recyclable components that minimize environmental impact. As the demand for sustainable living spaces grows, innovative design solutions continue to evolve, offering homeowners pathways to reduce their ecological footprint while enhancing their living environments.

Harnessing natural resources efficiently is a hallmark of eco-friendly home design. Passive solar design, an essential element, leverages sunlight for heating and lighting, reducing dependence on artificial sources. Strategic placement of windows and living spaces maximizes natural daylight, cutting energy use and creating inviting atmospheres. These thoughtful layouts show how design elements can work harmoniously with nature.

Choosing sustainable materials is pivotal in constructing or renovating a home with ecological responsibility in mind. Prioritizing locally sourced or rapidly renewable materials like bamboo or reclaimed wood supports reduced transportation emissions and promotes sustainable forestry practices. Likewise, recycled materials—when integrated seamlessly—lend an environmentally friendly and unique character to the home.

Energy efficiency extends further with the adoption of cutting-edge insulation techniques and eco-friendly heating systems. High-performance insulation maintains comfortable indoor temperatures, reducing the demand for energy-intensive systems. Additionally, incorporating heat recovery ventilation systems can significantly improve air quality while optimizing energy use, marrying comfort with conservation.

Green building certifications, such as LEED or BREEAM, provide frameworks for achieving various levels of sustainability in home design. These certifications guide homeowners and developers in integrating environmental considerations throughout the construction and operation phases. Meeting these standards ensures a commitment to ecological sensitivity and often results in long-term financial savings through enhanced energy efficiency.

In exploring eco-conscious home design, the potential for a harmonious living space becomes apparent—a place where elegance meets responsibility. As this journey unfolds, creative ideas and practical applications will emerge, illustrating diverse strategies to transform homes into sanctuaries of sustainability. Through thoughtful decisions and innovative features, the subsequent pages will delve deeper into how each element can contribute to a low-impact yet highly livable home.

Incorporating sustainable design into your home begins with a mindful evaluation of how each aspect of your living space interacts with the environment. This journey toward sustainability is guided by a commitment to choose materials and designs that offer both aesthetic appeal and environmental responsibility. By selecting low-impact, non-toxic building materials, you ensure that your home not only serves as a comfortable sanctuary but also aligns with ecological goals.

Opting for energy-efficient systems is another crucial step in minimizing a household's ecological impact. Installing advanced energy systems like solar panels and geothermal heating not only reduces reliance on fossil fuels but also contributes significantly to lowering utility costs over time. Such systems, while representing an initial investment, promise returns through reduced energy expenditure and enhanced property value.

Maximizing natural resources is central to eco-conscious design. Strategically placing windows and using materials that capitalize on natural ventilation can dramatically cut down on the need for artificial cooling or heating. These considerations extend to selecting thermal mass elements, such as brick or tile floors, which naturally regulate indoor temperatures by absorbing and releasing heat.

Water conservation plays an equally important role in eco-friendly home design. Integrating water-saving features like rainwater collection systems and greywater recycling can reduce fresh water use and help sustain a balanced ecosystem. These systems ensure that every drop is put to optimal use, reflecting a conscientious approach to resource management.

Beyond environmental benefits, these eco-friendly strategies offer a chance to enhance the quality of your life. Improved air quality and increased natural light foster healthier, more inviting living spaces. This balance of functionality and environmental sensitivity creates a home that resonates with tranquility and sustainability.

As these principles take root, they set the stage for exploring further innovations in sustainable design. The subsequent pages will delve into cutting-edge technologies and creative solutions that push the boundaries of what's possible in eco-conscious living, guiding homeowners toward a future where beauty and responsibility coexist harmoniously.

Creating an environmentally harmonious home involves integrating nature into design, fostering a seamless connection between indoor and outdoor spaces. Thoughtful design considerations can include utilizing large windows to frame natural vistas and inviting greenery into living areas. By blurring the boundaries between exterior and interior environments, you cultivate a tranquil ambiance that enhances both mental well-being and environmental awareness.

Fostering biodiversity in landscaping furthers eco-conscious practices. Selecting native plant species for your garden supports local ecosystems by providing essential habitats and food resources for wildlife. This not only enhances the ecological value of your property but also reduces the need for intensive water and pesticide use, aligning with sustainable gardening principles.

Implementing smart technology elevates home efficiency by monitoring and optimizing resource consumption. Intelligent irrigation systems, for instance, ensure that water use is precisely managed, adapting to weather conditions to prevent waste. Smart home energy systems can automate lighting and climate control, fine-tuning consumption to align with peak efficiency times. Such advancements illustrate the practical synergy between technology and sustainability, creating a more intelligent and responsive living environment.

Incorporating recycled or upcycled materials in design projects also reflects a commitment to sustainability. From reclaimed wood used in furniture to recycled glass in countertops, these materials infuse unique character into your home, each piece telling a story of renewal and creativity. Utilizing such resources minimizes environmental impact while showcasing innovative approaches to design and construction.

Encouraging the use of multipurpose spaces can optimize living areas, reducing the need for excessive construction and materials. Designing areas that can easily transition in function—from home office to guest room—not only conserves space but also simplifies living environments. This adaptability aligns with minimalist principles, emphasizing the need for fewer but more versatile spaces that cater to dynamically changing lifestyles.

As we've explored the multifaceted strategies in eco-friendly design, the path to creating a sustainable home becomes clear. This integration of aesthetics and ecological mindfulness results in spaces that nurture both inhabitants and the planet, embodying a commitment to responsible and inspired living.

Building a Community of Change

In the intricate tapestry of sustainable living, the power of community weaves individuals into a collective force capable of transformative change. The shared energy and commitment of like-minded individuals foster a dynamic exchange of ideas, strategies, and support, making the pursuit of sustainability both achievable and impactful. As we delve into this realm, we uncover the potential of collective action to amplify personal efforts and create lasting environmental change.

Engaging with your community offers a robust platform to propagate the principles of sustainable living. Local initiatives provide fertile ground for cultivating environmental awareness, from neighborhood clean-up drives to resource exchange programs. Participating in these activities enhances personal commitment to green practices and encourages others to join the movement, creating a ripple effect that extends beyond individual actions.

Advocacy within your immediate circle holds the power to influence broader environmental policies and practices. By voicing concerns at local meetings or joining eco-conscious groups, individuals can drive policy changes that align with sustainable goals. These efforts are not solitary; they harness collective voices to press for systemic changes that help shape a sustainable future for all.

Networking with like-minded individuals is central to building a resilient community of change-makers. Whether through joining local environmental clubs or participating in online forums, these connections serve as a resource for sharing experiences, gaining insights, and collectively tackling the environmental challenges at hand. These interactions foster a sense of solidarity and belonging, essential for sustaining motivation and commitment to green initiatives.

Education, as a vital component of this journey, bolsters community efforts by equipping individuals with the knowledge necessary to enact meaningful change. Workshops, seminars, and educational campaigns empower participants with practical tools and strategies for implementing sustainability in everyday life. This continuous learning keeps the community informed and adaptable to the evolving landscape of environmental practices.

As the dialogue grows and initiatives flourish, the importance of community-led action shines bright. It is this shared responsibility that paves the way for a more sustainable, equitable world, as collective efforts intertwine to fortify the fabric of sustainable living. Through engaged participation, education, and advocacy, communities can transform aspirations into reality, nurturing a legacy of environmental stewardship for future generations.

Building a sustainable community begins with recognizing the shared aspirations for a greener world. In neighborhoods, these aspirations take shape through initiatives like community gardens or compost stations, projects that offer practical solutions to reduce waste and boost food security. Through shared responsibilities, participants cultivate not only plants but also a stronger sense of connection and common purpose.

Engaging residents in educational programs is essential for fostering a culture of sustainability. By offering workshops that cover topics like renewable energy or waste reduction, communities empower their members with the skills and knowledge needed to implement environmentally friendly practices. These sessions not only enlighten but also inspire community-driven innovation, providing a platform for residents to exchange ideas and support one another.

Speaking up about local environmental issues in municipal forums allows communities to leverage their collective voices for systemic change. Outlining the benefits of sustainable practices to local councils can drive policy adjustments that prioritize ecological considerations, whether it's reducing plastic bag usage or increasing investment in green public spaces. This advocacy focuses not on confrontation but on collaboration with policymakers to achieve mutually beneficial outcomes.

Networking with organizations that have similar environmental goals extends the reach of community efforts. Forming alliances with these groups can open avenues for shared resources and expertise, ultimately magnifying the impact of local initiatives. By collaborating on larger projects, such as renewable energy installations or public transportation enhancements, communities can transform ambitious ideas into tangible, far-reaching improvements.

The reciprocal nature of community improvement ensures that as individuals contribute their skills and efforts, they receive support and motivation in return. This continuous cycle of giving and receiving builds resilience, positioning communities to better tackle environmental challenges. Through this collective energy, the community evolves into a dynamic force, constantly adapting and expanding its reach.

As communities continue to grow and evolve, the journey toward sustainability becomes not just a goal, but a way of life. With each iteration of these collective efforts, the fabric of the community strengthens, weaving new narratives of possibility and resilience, poised to embrace the challenges on the horizon.

Fostering a sustainable community demands a wholistic approach that seamlessly incorporates education, engagement, and empowerment. Initiating environmental clubs within schools or neighborhood groups can ignite interest and encourage participation across different age groups. These gatherings serve as platforms for exchanging actionable ideas, inspiring participants to explore practical ways they can contribute to sustainability daily. As interest broadens, the community becomes a hub of continuous learning and innovation.

Local initiatives such as skill-sharing workshops can be transformative. By inviting knowledgeable members to teach others—from composting techniques to energy-saving tips—communities nurture a sense of self-sufficiency and interconnectedness. These workshops become a fertile ground for creativity and problem-solving, encouraging everyone to take an active role in the movement toward sustainability.

Harnessing the prowess of digital tools can further amplify outreach and coordination. Creating online groups or forums allows community members to communicate swiftly, share resources, and update others on ongoing projects. These platforms can also serve as entry points for those new to sustainable practices, offering a welcoming environment where questions lead to shared growth.

Celebrating shared successes through community events strengthens bonds and reinforces commitment. Hosting an annual sustainability fair or expo can highlight achievements, showcasing everything from urban farming projects to waste reduction tactics. These occasions not only motivate participants to continue their efforts but attract new interest, expanding the reach and impact of community-driven endeavors.

The beauty of building a sustainable community lies in its cyclical reciprocity. Each contribution enriches the collective, while the strength of the collective emboldens individual action. This synergy ensures that even small actions, when multiplied across a community, can lead to significant and lasting change, transforming lives and local environments alike.

As this chapter concludes, it reinforces the message that the journey toward sustainability is a shared endeavor. By fostering a culture of learning and collaboration, communities become catalysts for change, emboldened by the knowledge that together, they hold the power to shape a viable and vibrant future for all.

The End